Alzheimer's
MY NEW LIFE BEGINS

TIMOTHY D. NORTON, ED.D.

Alzheimers: My New Life Begins

Copyright © 2017 by Dr. Timothy D. Norton. All rights reserved.

No part of this publication may be reproduced, stored in a retrieval system or transmitted in any way by any means, electronic, mechanical, photocopy, recording or otherwise without the prior permission of the author except as provided by USA copyright law.

The opinions expressed by the author are not necessarily those of Trilogy Christian Publishing, LLC.

Published by Trilogy Christian Publishing
c/o Trinity Broadcasting Network

PO Box A
Santa Ana, CA 92711

Trilogypub@tbn.org
714-425-4093

Book design copyright © 2017 by Trilogy Christian Publishing, LLC. All rights reserved.

Cover and Layout design by Kristen Polson

Published in the United States of America

ISBN: 9781640880047

Foreword

This chronicle represents only six months of my life. At 61 years of age, that is not representative of very much time; but, with respect to the continuance of my life, it represents its future. Alzheimer's has taken residence in my mind and will remain there until I leave it. These six months are presented to show the changes that have occurred. They are a revelation to me as much as they may be to you.

My new life has just begun. I am learning how to live and to maintain a sense of purpose in it. As with all of life's purposes, it is hoped that they will serve not only as an inspiration for the one experiencing them but also for others. This journey is intended to show my way. If my thoughts and experiences can help others in their journey, then my life will not have been traveled in vain. May God give to me and to them a purposeful journey and one that will safely lead us to His shore.

Dedication

This book is dedicated to my family - Gary and Barbara, Sheri and Arthur, Tonya and Butch, Tim and Molly, Anne and Marvin, and my six grand-children – Mackenzie, Liam, Keegan, Jazmine, Matthew, and Joshua - as well as to my friends who have always been a major part of my life. Their commitment to our love and friendship will comfort and guide me through this new path in God's will. I thank them for always being there.

Thanksgiving Day, November 24

Yesterday, I found out from my doctor that I have a type of dementia. I asked him how many types of dementia there are and he told me that there were a number of them and that he believed I had the most common – Alzheimer's. I suggested since both my mother and uncle had had Alzheimer's, that would add to the likelihood of my having it. He indicated that would probably be the case.

He then referred me to a neuropsychologist to have some further tests taken in order to confirm his diagnosis. He said it would probably take a couple of months to get an appointment with the specialist.

Although I could hear the compassion in his voice – after literally changing my life – all he could do was give me some pills.

November 26

The new felt fear seems odd to me. Having lived by myself for so many years and now feeling uncomfortable alone is a strange and uneasy feeling. It's not me, but it seems to be becoming me. Nothing has really changed. I have always enjoyed the singleness of the evening. Working, reading, watching some TV, and enjoying the presence of Cody, my dog, I never felt fear. But that seems to be then, and this is now. What a very big difference a 'feeling' can make.

December 27

It's difficult to know when to tell them. I don't see the specialist for another month. I don't know if I will get his results right away or even until another month after that. Being in town visiting my two children, their spouses, and my six grandchildren, all of whom live in York, Pennsylvania, makes it easier to share. The problem is that I don't know the extent of the disease or the time frames for its progression. That is something that the specialist will need to tell me. The dilemma is whether it is better to tell them face-to-face or from a distance. I don't want to return home leaving them with too many unanswered questions; but, I also don't want to wait and then have the 'telling' come across as being too impersonal. I leave in a few more days; I guess the decision will definitely be made by then.

January 3

I have always been a late-night person. Going to the grocery store at 1:00 or 2:00 a.m. was not unusual for me, as I was never concerned about the night. I am finding now that the evening presents a concern. Not that I am afraid of the night, but that I am afraid that I might not remember my way in the night. I now wonder, what if I am on my way home and I forget how to get there? Would I be able to find the way home in the darkness? When I travel on the roads with an abundance of lighting, I am not as concerned. But, in Tulsa, we have many roads that are not very well lit. If I were to break down or make a wrong turn, could I see my way through or would I get lost?

January 7

Today was an adverse Alzheimer's day. The previous three days had been wonderful. I was able to drive to wherever I wanted to go without thinking about how to get there. I didn't feel the fear that I do some days. I even briefly wondered if I had Alzheimer's. But today it all came back. I had the fear. I had to 'think' about where I was driving. I knew for sure that I had the disease. I suppose that my life will be topsy-turvy until I no longer can separate it from the consequences of the disease. It is interesting to imagine that my body will determine what I can and cannot think. How far away that day is, I do not know. But I must live as if it will never come in order to live my life now.

January 8

I have spent the day feeling the 'fear,' and it suddenly dawned on me that the Lord has not given us a spirit of fear. I know certain aspects of the disease will affect me, but I am convinced that the fear can be overcome with the help of the Lord. My mind may change, but does my spirit have to join it? I don't think so. Tonight, I will remember the words of the Lord and put them to the test. I believe that He will be faithful and that the fear will subside and eventually leave me. Not because the disease has changed, but because my faith has changed.

January 9

Today was the first day back from Christmas break for the faculty. We had a full-day session with a guest speaker and breakouts to evaluate the topics shared. I would estimate that at least 150 faculty and additional support personnel were in attendance. We were separated into tables of eight, with each table having an individual who was responsible to lead the discussions after each of the speaker's presentations. I was the leader at my table.

The intellectual banter and investigative spirit was present as we sought for new ways to share the knowledge in each of our disciplines. As the day came to an end, I realized that this kind of activity, which has been part of my life for over 35 years, may soon come to a close. The colleagues and their friendships will be lost to me. My fond memories will be as absent as I will be. Hopefully, though I will not remember, some will.

January 13

This morning was a casual one, so I went to my closet to pick out a sweatshirt. I went to grab one and noticed that my argyle sweater that I had worn yesterday was on the top of the pile. I keep my sweaters in my dresser in my bedroom. Realizing that I had put it in the wrong place the night before made me laugh as it brought to mind my time with my mother just before she passed last May. She also had Alzheimer's. With the four siblings, we each had taken different times in the year to have her visit with us. Being a college professor, I always had her during the summer months when I did not teach full time.

I can remember her putting things in all kinds of places and me 'finding' them. Remembering her time with me and the joy that we had together helps me to understand better this time in my life. This is just another way for me to experience my life and to see the joy in it when it can be seen. My mother taught me that in so many ways, and she is still teaching me today.

January 18

How many times can I forget? As many times as there are moments in a day. Regrettably, since this statement is true, there is one place I have been able to go for help with this cumbersome problem – my cell phone. Where else can I repeatedly refer for answers to the variety of questions that arise during the day? No matter how many times I need to know when something is supposed to occur, or when others are expecting me, my cell phone never seems to be irritated by my continued requests. It 'answers the call' every time without criticism or complaint. Its patience is unending, and its assurance ever available.

Though the help of a friend or loved one is irreplaceable, their patience can have limits. Such a limitation is never found with my cell phone. It is accurate, comforting, and most of all, available for what I need and doesn't mind if I need it often. It may not be man's best friend, but for me, it may end up being my most accessible best friend.

January 21

A letter arrived from the law office handling my mother's financial portfolio. The figures were all presented and the totals given. How interesting to think that an entire life's financial holdings can be summarized in just a few statements and listings. Her life was more than that. She had married three times and raised four children. At the end, she showed me how to live a life with Alzheimer's. I think of her as I am experiencing my walk and remember her laughter and grace. I can only hope that when I get to the point of complete envelopment by the disease, I will live the rest of my life as she did, reflecting strength and holding close all whom she loved.

January 22

I had not planned on telling the family until I had my appointment with the specialist. However, I had a conversation with my sister, Sheri, and it led to my having to share with her my condition. As we talked about the topic, I had an overwhelming feeling that a dark cloud was covering my thoughts. How to tell your sister that her brother may one day not even know who she is or how much she means to him.

I have another sister, Tonya, and a brother, Gary, and for any of us to live our lives without the other would be a contemplation none of us would have wanted to consider. Death does come to each of us, but 'present' separation is never imagined. Though one day I may forget, the feelings we each have shared over a lifetime are part of what makes us who we are.

January 25

In the evening before I go to bed, I hang up the clothes that I have had on throughout the day. That's what I do. This particular evening was no exception, at least that was what I thought. The next morning as I was getting dressed, I noticed that my shirt and the shirt hanger were still on the bed. I had hung up my pants from the night before, but not the shirt. I had gotten the hanger out of the closet in order to hang up the shirt, but had not done so. I realized that although I thought it had been done, I just didn't do it. The shirt and the hanger had been on the end of the bed all night, and I had not noticed or felt like I had not completed my evening task. Though not a major problem, this was the first time that something that I had not done remained undone without my notice.

It reminded me of the times when my mother would leave things undone and I would gently remind her to do them. I had no one to remind me. Just as it was odd for me to see what I had not done, so it must have been hard for Mom to see the same in her actions. Though the disease will separate me from some, it can bring memories that make me feel closer to others. This is a small joy in the midst of great change.

January 27

I just had a little bit of trouble finding a gas station. This particular station has non-ethanol gasoline. I like to fill my tank with that type of gas. It is just around the corner from my house, but I couldn't find it. In Tulsa, all the main roads are set in squared blocks, a mile apart from East to West and also North to South. Once you know where a place is, it is easy to find again. The problem is that if you have a corner in mind and you are wrong regarding its location, there are no particular driving differences in order to find where that corner is actually located. The only way is to travel the road's square miles until you happen to run into it.

It's a great layout as long as you know where the place you are looking for is and where you are going. But if you don't, all the intersections seem the same. At least, they do when you have memory challenges with your thinking. I finally stumbled onto the place for which I was searching. Of course, once found, I knew exactly where it had been all along. I just couldn't find it until I had found it. That may sound odd, but that is how one begins to think when met with Alzheimer's.

January 31

All day testing! Who could ask for more? Those were my thoughts when my primary care physician scheduled me for testing to verify his belief that I had Alzheimer's. The appointment began at 8:00 a.m. and finished at 3:45 p.m. that afternoon. By lunch, I could not remember the last time I had felt so brain-dead. I suppose working on the concluding part of my dissertation may have been close, but I am not sure. By the end of the day, I had experienced practically every kind of brain taxing test one could imagine. Mathematics, grammar, word problems, general concepts, playing with blocks, colors, sizes, memory lists, general knowledge, specific thinking ideas on particular subjects and concepts, and many other kinds of 'thought' things. We finally ended with a 344-question questionnaire on practically every kind of knowledge and conceptualization imaginable. It then took another hour for the specialist, who had not been administering the tests, to review the information in order to share it with me.

I sat in the testing area waiting for his time with me. When he finally got there, he indicated that I needed to check with my primary physician to see if he wanted to share the test results with me or whether he wanted the specialist to do it. After almost eight hours of testing and waiting, I was now going to need to check and see which doctor was to share the information with me. Of course, that would mean, once I knew who I was to meet with, setting up another appointment before I would know the results. At that point, he indicated that the testing had gone well and sent me on my way.

Going home, I thought about the day and the reason for it. How unimaginable was the idea that what I had just taken only represented a few hours in my life, but what I had just completed would be the predictor of the remaining years of my life to come.

February 5

I have, for most of my adult life, had to work to maintain a healthy weight. Not in the obese sense, but just as a normal fellow who likes to eat. That is beginning to change. I still love to eat, but I find myself unintentionally eating less. Some might think that this is a great thing, especially if they have struggled with weight in the past. However, in my case, it is not due to dieting, but to the lack of a desire to eat as much as I used to. I just find food less inviting. I'm not sure if this is a good or bad thing. In the long run, it may mean nothing, as long as it does not continue. If it does, it may mean that I will have to 'make myself' eat more. Considering my life up to this point, I would have never thought that this would ever be a problem with which I would need to deal.

February 6

I am living my life. I am not 'in a life' of Alzheimer's. Though my mind is beginning to change, it is still 'my' mind. We all will die one day. That day is never known. The day does not change because of a disease. The Lord numbers all of our days, and we must fulfill each one. Alzheimer's may be the 'way' my life ends, but it does not have control over my life. God's will always supersedes any other means of charting our days. Why? Because He desires to live eternally with us, and 'death' serves as the door of entrance to that life. Just like the first time you leave home, it's a little scary. Leaving this life can be a little scary, too. But when you leave home your parents tell you that you will be alright. God does the same in that He says that the death of the saint is precious in His eyes.

He is watching and He is waiting.

February 7

Have you ever realized that something that you thought was wrong was actually right? As a college professor, my main emphasis is to help people learn to think correctly about whatever they are trying to think about. This evening, I experienced thinking wrongly when I was intentionally trying to think rightly.

I was ironing a shirt. When I was done, in order to put the iron back in its place, I looked up at the series of four cabinet doors over the washer and dryer in my utility room. I opened one cabinet door and placed the iron in it. I immediately thought that I had put the iron in the wrong place and removed it. I then opened each cabinet door, surveyed the contents, and then closed it. I was unable to figure out which cabinet was the right one. After doing this several times, it finally dawned on me that the first cabinet, the one that I had originally chosen, was actually the right place for the iron.

One interesting thing about thinking is, until you show your mind that it is not thinking correctly, it always assumes that it already is. The problem with Alzheimer's is that it sometimes takes a while for you to realize you are thinking wrongly, and then even longer before you realize that you have not been thinking rightly all along. This is where patience checks in, both for the one with the disease, and more importantly, for the one who cares.

February 9

I am dying. Very few people get to so closely identify with that phrase. We all know that we will die, but I not only know that I will die; I know that I am dying. My life may be 'cut short' by Alzheimer's, but my death 'is prolonged' by it. Usually, when one knows that they are dying, death is imminent. For me, Alzheimer's death is a journey, as it has already confirmed its presence and yet hasn't taken me. I can live in the midst of my own death. For every moment that I experience is part of my living and part of my dying. To remember yesterday's events is to also realize that they will be the present memories of me when I pass. It makes life and death more of a singular event in the totality of being a person. Life is enriched when you know its ending is near. Death is comfortable when you have 'lived' with it awhile. The dichotomy of their differences fades in the realization of their continuance.

February 11

As a graduate professor, I teach classes in a modular format. This means that my students come into town and have class for three days - on Thursday from 5:00 p.m. to 9:00 p.m. and on Friday and Saturday from 8:00 a.m. to 5:00 p.m. I was scheduled to teach a doctoral level course in the Governance and History of Colleges and Higher Education. This would be the first course that I would teach since my primary physician had indicated that he thought I had Alzheimer's. I wondered if my mind would be able to 'teach' at a doctoral level or if I would forget the information I had to present. I also was concerned that I would be unable to interact with these students as they would expect.

The class began, and I did what I usually do and the students gave no indications that I was not being the teacher that I should be and that they expected. I had some concern as they presented their last oral presentations on the research topic assigned in the class. It involved the history of higher education in America. As they presented, there were a number of facts and situations upon which I needed to comment. I then concluded the class and the students thanked me for an enjoyable learning experience. This simply shows that when you put your trust in the Lord, He will see you through. Yet, at some point, my abilities may change, and if they do, I will need to be able to face that reality.

February 13

At age 61, I did not think that I qualified for anything 'younger' anymore. But I was wrong. It seems that I fit into the 'younger-onset' Alzheimer's category. This group is comprised of 200,000 out of the 5.5 million people in America with Alzheimer's. The remaining 5.3 million are those who are 65 and older. I am .0005% of the 200,000 in the younger category. Everyone wants to feel like they fit into a unique group, but sometimes the honor is not one we would have chosen for ourselves.

Though younger, being in a statistically smaller group does not prevent me from having the same issues with the disease. My memory will still fade and my abilities lessen. I will just have these things happen sooner, rather than later, as I am growing older. I may live the same number of years as others diagnosed later in life, but I will still have the distinction of having 'died too soon.' Irony sometimes plays a part in most of our lives, but when centered on the conclusion of our life, it seems even more bitter.

February 17

Tonight, I am very tired, and that does not help my ability to think. Like everyone else in the world, I have been tired. This tired, though, is not the same. It is one in which I can't seem to think like I would normally be able to. I want to think, but my mind won't do it. The feeling is strange in that I can't make myself work past it. Having been a student for many years, I know how to make myself think when it is late at night and I have to finish a paper or prepare for a test. Every student has sensed that need and been able to press through. This evening, as I am writing this, I pause more frequently than usual. The frustration for me as a professor is that what one does naturally, tonight is unnatural. Maybe tomorrow will be better. That is what we all hope for. But, when tomorrow is another day with Alzheimer's, you never know.

February 18

Feeling sick to my stomach and wanting to throw up seems to be a common experience with my Alzheimer's. I don't know if it is 'normal' or just unique to me. It doesn't happen every day, but it is frequent enough for me to consider it as part of my illness. I am able to function but carry with me the perspective of this unsettling condition. It does rob me of the 'anticipation of certain moments' throughout the day but must be overcome in order for me to not miss the 'experiencing of each moment.' For those who have lived their entire life with a major illness, this may not be unique. For me, however, everything associated with this disease is new.

February 19

This is my 'once' and it's ok. I have been a little depressed thinking about the conclusion of my life. It seems premature to me. I have thought that this can't be the way I will go. It was never in my plan. Death was part of the plan, as it is inevitable, but Alzheimer's wasn't. I knew that something would take me, but I thought it would be old-age, not what some may call 'premature death.' However, if you consider that He holds all things in His hands and that He is sovereign, then this is not premature and it is His plan.

His Word declares that, "It is appointed unto man once to die." I have one appointment with death. That appointment has been preordained before the beginning of time. The cause has also been predetermined. I am in His hands, not the hands of the disease. As with everyone else, I am on my way to 'my way' to die. I may know that it is closer than I thought, but that does not change the fact that this way has always been my appointed 'once' to die.

February 20

I had a thought in mind. I just came from the den. Figured I would write about it. Just can't remember what it was. I have a few suggested Alzheimer's writings that I had previously put on a 'to do list' here in my home office. Looking at them, they don't seem to be good topics. One was about my concern with having one of my university classes videotaped and my not remembering all the course topic information. Another was creating 'a list' of things that I forget in order to write about them. Neither of these sounds interesting right now. They may be tomorrow, but they aren't now.

The idea that the 'illness' affects my mood is troublesome to me. Like most people know, emotions are not always the best directors of action. We are taught to control them, not that we should let them control us. I have never been a person who had mood swings, but some of the feelings I am beginning to experience are troublesome to me. They are a difference that I am not sure that I will be able to control.

February 27

This morning I had to accomplish a number of things at my university office. While there, I had a sense of uneasiness. I also did not feel well as I was nauseous and had a strange sense of loneliness. I had this before at home, but never at work. Although I was not well, I still had things I had to accomplish that were part of my job, so I stayed.

In the afternoon, I had a committee meeting to go to. I thought that it was not going to be easy, as I still felt the way I had earlier. Surprisingly, the sensations of nausea and loneliness faded and things went well. I interacted as I should have as a faculty member. I came home from work and the sensations of nausea and loneliness returned.

Since I have lived alone for a while, I am beginning to realize that Alzheimer's may have some impact on the new feelings of loneliness and physical discomfort I am having. I have never been a back and forth kind of person. I don't know if the disease can affect people that way. I now have another question for my doctor the next time I see him. It is interesting to have a disease that continually affords new revelations daily.

February 25

I have made a decision. I believe that part of the problem with the 'fear' is that since I am not used to it, I assumed that it was in control due to the disease. Because of this thinking, I had begun to limit my solo trips to places in the mid to late evenings, especially after dark. Tonight, I determined that as long as I have any mental abilities, I, and not Alzheimer's, will be in control. This is not foolish thinking but logical. There is never a reason to surrender until you have been completely overtaken. Opportunity does not guarantee success. It just allows the one trying, even if just for a brief moment, to feel victorious.

February 26

I had taken my dress shoes to the shoe shop to have them shined. It was the next day, and I dressed for work and put on my tennis shoes. I went to the cobbler and, while there, traded the tennis shoes for the dress ones. The cobbler put the tennis shoes in a plastic bag, and I put them in the back of my car.

The next day, Saturday, I spent most of the day at home in my slippers. When it was time to go out to dinner, I went to put on my tennis shoes. They were not in my closet. I looked for them throughout the house but could not find them. I searched the house several times, including looking under the beds and in all the different bedroom closets. I still could not find them. Where would I have left them? It all made no sense. Finally, I thought that I may have, for some reason or another, left them in my car. I went out to the garage and looked in the front and backseats of the car. Just behind the drivers' seat was the bag from the cobblers. I immediately realized why it was there. I knew that I had had my dress shoes repaired and that I had spent the previous day in my tennis shoes.

Though I felt relieved, I knew that this was one more instance where my 'memory' was not with me. I had to find it. Sometimes one does not find the things one is looking for. I do not look forward to that day.

February 28

Yesterday, I had an appointment with my primary care physician to discuss the full-day testing results.

The report from the neuropsychologist indicated that I had "early onset dementia of the Alzheimer's type."

The main question has now been answered.

It seems that when one's 'present' changes, harder questions about one's future will then need to be asked.

March 4

Today was a 'clear' day. I had no issues remembering anything. When I talked with people, I felt inwardly confident. There was no concern that the conversation would politely switch to something that I should know but wouldn't remember. I was just like the old Tim. It is wonderful to be able to believe in your own abilities. Not in a prideful way, but with appropriate confidence. Not only do you momentarily believe, but you sense the ease in others as you are the person they believe that you are. The old Tim is not 'old' to them, it is still who they think that I am. It's not pretending, it's being 'me.' Yes, today was a clear day, but I know that it won't last forever.

March 5

Conversations are interesting things everyone shares, but they don't always serve to reveal. This is particularly the case if one has something to hide. I do. I don't want anyone to know what I am experiencing until I have finished what I am writing. That way they can read my thoughts and not just conclude their own. I wonder if I am making mistakes and they are thinking about them without saying anything to me. 'Being concerned' is becoming an everyday feeling. Not that others are intentionally making me feel that way; I am making me feel that way, as I wonder if I have forgotten something or have I made it obvious that I am not remembering.

Double-checking yourself is what we sometimes do when conversing with others. We check to see if we are following the conversation and not misinterpreting comments. But when you double-check yourself because you are not sure if what you're saying is revealing too much about you, it's like being on ice in regular shoes – you have to walk very carefully to make sure you don't slip.

March 6

I just noticed the empty heating pad box. This, of course, means that I must have used the heating pad recently and did not put it back in the box. But when did I use it, and where is the pad now? This type of situation may be typical for many, but with me there is a difference. It's not just the two questions that I must answer; I also must 'find' the ability to answer them. Great questions, but did I really use the heating pad, and if so, where is it?

The obvious sign that I must have used it is also the obvious indicator that I don't remember ever using it. Then I must go through the searching of my mind to first confirm that I used it and then to remember why I used it. Even though I live alone, my mind is not totally convinced that 'I' misplaced it. Maybe it's just an empty box. But I know better, so I begin to 'try' to bring the information to my memory.

Imagine looking at a blank chalkboard and trying to remember the math problem that was last covered in the class you took a week ago. You would first have to remember when the class was, where you sat in the class, what you were trying to learn, how it was presented, what classwork exercises you did, and did you actually understand them. If you look at that from the viewpoint of needing to answer a similar step-by-step process to remember something, it can be difficult.

Just as with the math problem, you can't skip a step. If I lose a step or forget one, the idea may not return. An additional problem is that you don't have a textbook that gives you the steps, so the ones that worked last time may not work this time. This time they worked. I remembered and realized that I had used the heating pad to ease my back discomfort last night and had left it in the study. I went to the study, and there it was plugged into the wall behind my chair. Even if it had been there for several days, it would not have been an issue. But having not made that choice myself, it is one more time when the disease is deciding for me.

March 7

A colleague, who had come into town because she was the Chair of a student's dissertation defense, made an interesting comment to me. She noticed that in our conversations I had several times of memory lapse, and she attributed them to my being a 'little fatigued.' Because she had no knowledge of what to connect it to, she assumed that it was just normal memory loss from tiredness. We all have that from time to time. I made no comment and the conversation changed to something else. No doubt, I had been tired, and also no doubt that I had the memory loss.

This was the first time, at least to me, that someone had made the memory loss and tiredness connection. Though I had noticed, now someone else had also noticed. There are no intended secrets, but neither are there any revealing confessions. A crack in the wall had been seen. I believed that this time I would be safe from further inquiries. After all, at my age, everyone has some memory issues. How quickly will the next time occur? When will the cracks become larger? Those will be my continued unanswered questions.

March 8

I am the co-faculty sponsor for an international education honor society in the College of Education. Tonight, we had an induction for new members. I knew that there would be a series of introductions of the faculty and students who would be assisting in the induction. I would be introducing my colleagues who had come to help. There were a total of twelve of them. When it came time to introduce them, I had no name list as these were people I knew very well. I was doing just fine until I got to the last faculty member, who was also going to be the new incoming President of our college chapter.

As the co-faculty sponsor, the other sponsor and I had decided that this faculty member would serve in this position. I called her by a different though similar first name and then called her last name using the honorific 'doctor.' I immediately cautiously changed that only to realize that I had gotten the 'doctor' part right. I eventually fell upon both the correct first and last name and presented her again, including the doctor title. I used a little bit of humor to cover the mistake and it was treated as the kind of mistake that could be accidentally committed. I, however, knew the difference. After the meeting, I apologized to the professor, and she laughed.

No one knew the real reason for my mistake. They just thought that it was one of those things that happens in public speaking situations. I was grateful for her 'forgiveness' but troubled by this latest concern. Eventually, there will be too many of these situations that an apology will not work. At some point, the day will come, I will tell them, and the answer to my concern will become evident.

March 9

"You are wise beyond all measure and Your ways are perfect." This was the closing confession of my prayers to You this night. I know that I am in the center of Your will.

Man's sin opened the door, but God's will rules the day. I am not in doubt. I walk this road because You have required it of me. Only You can deliver me. There is currently no cure, but Your purpose still remains. Others may believe that the illness has its way. I believe that You are the Way. Though I walk through the valley of the shadow of death, I will fear no evil. Your comfort in the midst of Your will shall be my testimony. Others may walk this path alone, but for me, You are with me and will see me through to the end. I can believe no other and I can confess no less.

March 10

The ending has begun. Yesterday, I had two conversations at work, one with the Chair of the Department and the other with the Dean. For the first I was asked to meet, the second, I suggested the meeting. In my first meeting, the Chair had mentioned that the Dean had told him how I had not remembered a faculty member's name at the KDP induction. He had not been able to be there, so I confirmed her perspective on the evening. The Chair reminded me that he and I had previously discussed my memory issues. He mentioned that other faculty had brought their concerns to him and wondered if I had any new information on the subject. I told him that I appreciated the others concerns and shared that my doctor had tested me and I asked if I could wait to cover things until the end of the semester. He agreed. I also asked if he would mind if I went ahead and spoke to the Dean.

I went to the Dean's office, and she shared her concerns regarding the previous evening. I explained to her the testing that had occurred and asked her if I could delay the conversation until the end of the semester. She, very graciously, told me that if she ever put me in a situation where my memory issues might prove uncomfortable, please let her know and she would rearrange things. I told her I appreciated very much her understanding and would keep her informed.

Though I had received a report from the doctor, I did not want to cover it at this point, as I had not yet had an opportunity to tell my family. I did not want them to think that they might have been the last to know. My discussion of the particulars would not have changed the conclusion of my discussion with my bosses, but it could have had a very significant impact on my family. Having several groups of people with different needs and attachments to my story makes it difficult, especially when dealing with something that you cannot control becomes the very reason why you must control it.

March 12

There are two sides to every coin. Depending on which side you see as you are holding it in your hand, it shows you either heads or tails. Each of us has the same configuration, the person that others see and the person that only we see. When illness changes the outer image, it is harder for others to see the inner image of you that remains hidden.

Alzheimer's is a disease that hides the person inside, both from others and from the person themselves. Once lost, the person becomes more difficult to find. It isn't easy for the one with the disease or for those who are trying to help. Both are looking for the same 'person,' but neither can help the other find him.

March 13

Today, I told my children, Tim and Anne, about my Alzheimer's. Since neither one of them was home when I called, I left a message. Tim was the first to call me back. He was very concerned, and we talked about the situation. I shared how I would be depending upon him, as he is a lawyer. He brought up some of the 'lawyer' type things we needed to discuss, and as he did so, he softly broke into tears. He mentioned how this kind of thing was so much easier with others but so difficult with his own Dad. I smiled a little bit thinking of my son, the lawyer, and all of the stereotyping that goes with that, tearing up while talking with his Dad about those typical things he talks about with others. His tears brought tears to my eyes, and we softly cried together as we continued to discuss the other 'lawyer' type things. He and I had our time, father and son.

Anne and I talked that afternoon. She indicated to me that she would have a room ready if I ever needed one. We discussed the future and what could happen and how we would all make it through. Later, Marvin, her husband, called and also mentioned that they would have a place for me when needed. He further indicated that he expected that he would need to have a place for Cody, my dog. It is amazing when God forms a family, how willing they are to play a part in making that family the best it can be. Today, my children have made that a reality.

March 15

I was looking for some assistance in understanding my disease. I went to the Oklahoma Alzheimer's Association website. To my surprise, its office is located in the CityPlex Towers. These towers are owned by Oral Roberts University and are across the street from the campus. It was nice that, when I called, they confirmed that they were there to help in any way they could. I felt as if I was already connected to someone who knew about my disease. It's like when you find out as a freshman in college that your roommate is from the same town as you. There is a natural connection which leads to mutual comradery. You easily walk through things together. I know that what I am saying may be only an imagined closeness, but with this illness, imagination may be one of the best defenses. I know that all things work together for good, but it is nice, when in the wilderness, God has His oasis.

March 16

Byron, my friend from Canada, called today. He and I had rooms beside each other when we were in the dorms during our undergraduate education at Oral Roberts University. We have been friends ever since, and he and his three sisters, Jill, Holly, and Nancy, and I talk on occasion. I had called him earlier and left a message regarding my condition.

As we talked, I could hear their concern and also felt their encouragement to trust in the Lord for healing. After a while, they prayed for me. Byron had left a phone message earlier indicating that they wanted me to join them in The Lord's Supper that evening. I had gotten the elements for me, and we all rejoiced together in the celebration of His sacrifice and resurrection.

It is wonderful when those whom you love also love you. Their friendship always helps you to stand in whatever you are going through. Your life and theirs complement and support one another. They will remain friends forever in this life, but more importantly, in the life to come.

March 17

Alzheimer's not only changes your mind, it changes your schedule. When I first started writing these vignettes, I would jot down a few lines on a piece of note paper and then, later in the day or evening, complete my thoughts. I did this until recently. Now I have found that I need to go ahead and write about the topic while it is not only fresh in my mind but literally 'still' in my mind. The process has changed. My mind does not keep my thoughts as well as it used to. That is amazing for one who has always been the 'go to' guy for 'What was it that we decided last time?'

Things change and so do you, even when you don't consciously initiate that change. I think that is the hardest part of the disease. You don't always know when things are going to change, and you can't prepare yourself to 'go with it.' It makes the change and demands that you follow. Following its lead, when you don't know the change has been made, is not easy.

March 18

Today, I prepared for the end of my life. At least that is what it is called. My son asked me what I had or had not done in preparation for the conclusion of work and life. He sent me an email querying me regarding 'End of Life Planning documents' - A Living Will and a POA, Retirement/Resignation, STD/LTD benefit plans, Medicaid Planning, Retirement Planning, Retirement location or facility, and other relevant considerations. Though he is doing the 'right' thing as a good lawyer should do, I know that neither of us sees this as something either one of us wants to do.

There are times that a son has to be a lawyer, and there are times that a dad must be a client. Neither of us likes it, but it is what is best. Imagine, that thought is usually what parents have to think when disciplining a child. Today, it has now become the thought a child must think when blessing a parent.

March 19

My pants in the wrong place in the closet. An empty heating pad box. Putting on tennis shoes instead of dress shoes. Humor, a creative necessity. We all have those moments when we see humor in something. It is in human nature and part of human need. We can't truly live life to the fullest without it. God has made us to need humor. He has put humor in the world through so many of the humorous things His other living creatures do. He has also given it to man as seen by the way we think and live. Life without humor is barely life at all. Humor is not a feeling; it is a living expression of our very being. It does not fade as we do. It continues through each stage of our life. Only when we become discouraged do we begin to lose our sense of humor. We must guard against this, as God has given humor to us as a shelter in the storm.

March 20

I am beginning to relive my mother's life. When she would stay with me for the summer, she would many times start something and then leave it without completely finishing it. I am still met with that surprise. I have found dishes in the dishwasher after I had completely emptied it. Seen shirts in my walk-in closet hanging across on the other side with my pants. Plugged in the vacuum in the den when I wanted to vacuum another room. I use a CPAP machine that needs to be filled with water each night. I think it is full and don't know until the next morning that I forgot.

Some of these types of little forgetful things may seem normal to you as you may have done something similar. The difference is that when you see what you have done, your memory remembers how and why it happened. My memory is completely void of the incident, and if I did not live alone, I would be sure that someone else had done the forgetting. My memory is not faded or unsure; it remains void for those occurrences. They say that 'Life Happens;' for me, it sometimes doesn't.

March 21

Frustration, irritation, and justification. This trilogy seems to be surfacing too often when I am having interactions with others. I am beginning to realize that I 'can't' remember some things. This is frustrating. I defend this by being irritated with those who don't seem to me to understand my frustration. And I qualify my actions with justifications that present my perspective as the most acceptable. This trilogy does nothing to calm the situation but only to inflame it. Yet, I feel that I must do this because I can't solve these problems as I can't always 'think' what is the best way to resolve them. And, as always, when I lash out at others, I have only made the situation worse. Especially when these others are the ones that you need and they want to help. It is not a desire to win one's way; it is a fear of losing one's way.

March 22

We all want to go to heaven. That's what we are taught from a very early age. We don't really wonder how and when, we just want to go. One day, for most, it just happens. For me, I do wonder, as I now have the 'how' and that my 'when' is definitely on the way.

Usually, a trip becomes a reality when you begin to contemplate the how and when. As children, we start to get excited when we know that we can begin to think and talk about the how and when. The family changes their usual activities in anticipation of the how and when. Schedules alter, people are told, plans are made, and times are set. Excitement becomes the daily feeling. It's almost time, and the trip will begin.

I can now think that way. I must plan. There are people to thank, places to see, times to be remembered, and loves to be cherished. I am fortunate, as I know that I must do these things now. My trip must be planned, and I must anticipate its 'how and when.' In so doing, my life will continue to be a celebration of how's and when's to come and not of things that never will be. You can't ask for more than that!

March 23

She returned a few days ago. She lives under the covering of my backyard porch on a small shelf. She usually sits in her nest throughout the Spring and guards her young until they take their first flight. Occasionally, we 'talk' together, and she looks very intently at me. I don't know when it all started, but I am glad it continues. It's these kinds of simple things that tend to fill one's memories of life.

The fact that I have been able, without even trying, to affect the continuance of her life, enriches mine. I have pondered her absence and hoped that she will return. I have anticipated, with joy, that return. And I hope that in the future, we will once again see each other. I have wondered, when I am not here and if she is, will the next owner see what I see! One of the greatest mysteries in life is that when you think that you are being a blessing, you discover that in so doing, you are the one blessed.

March 24

My life is not an evolving sense of history, but a directed one that He has for me as part of His creation. There is no doubt that others believe that they just 'are' and that all of life is a conglomeration of events that then concludes as their 'life lived.' The past, present, and future are not theirs, but they are part of them. For both beliefs, there is an essence of 'living' within situations that envelope them. For each, there are different authors of those situations. For one, the author is eternal, for the other, the author is chance. One is directional, the other is positional. One has a future place, the other has no conclusion, it just ends.

When you consider these differences, why are the lives of people lived the same? How can one person of one persuasion have the same illness as a person of a different persuasion? If one believes in the eternal and the other does not, why would their actual living have the same experience? How can one life, which is subject to His direction, still experience the same illness as one who does not follow His direction? The answer is simple. For the one, the illness is giving an opportunity for the acknowledgement of praise to Him through the person's life. For the other, life is subject to the situations of this evolved world and the person must endure his life. To live through or to endure one's life, that is the question!

March 25

Memories, the current thoughts of thoughts passed by. We all live with them, and they make our living a remembrance. When they fade, it is not that they have just gone, but part of who we are has gone. When we remember, we bring back to life part of our life which lays the reason for our continued life. When we can't remember, we not only lose our past but we also lose our reason for the future. Memory serves as the foundation for who and what we are and why we do what we do. Alzheimer's steals that memory and provides no substitute. We ask, and we no longer hear an answer. We look and eventually do not find. We seek and there is nowhere to go.

March 26

I was remarking to a friend how I had remembered in our conversation something that, earlier in the day, I could not even begin to remember. It helped me to see that things that I fail to remember at one point sometimes reappear in my memory. They are gone to me and then, once again, become a part of me. I do not know if these same memories will continue to play disappearing and reappearing roles. I do not know if future memories will do the same. I am at their beck and call; they are no longer at mine.

Before Alzheimer's, I had variations in my memory just like everyone else. Some things stayed, and others came and went. It took only a slight contemplation and I could recall them and place them where they could not be forgotten. I was master of my own memory. Now I am not. Things come and go as they will, and I try to corral them in vain. One moment they are there, and then they are not. Occasionally, they reappear, and at other times, they just stay away. My mind and its thoughts are now part of the disease, and my dominion has been diminished.

March 27

God makes missionaries and then gives them a 'field.' God allows sin and then gives a 'savior.' God afflicts men and then gives them 'deliverance.' My God is faithful to Himself and therefore faithful to me. My affliction, even though it may be unto death, is present to show God's healing. My sin has allowed my affliction. His sacrifice will allow my healing.

Who can know the plans of the Lord? Who can see His purposes? Only those who are called by His name. Only those who He gives eyes to see and ears to hear. Only those whose hearts He has turned toward Him. I do not know because I know, I know because I am known. My affliction, though ever present to me, is just a moment for Him. I languish in my death, He prepares for my eternal life. I think of my world, He welcomes me to His. I remember my present, He establishes my future.

I do not say this in despair; I say it in the truth that He is and will ever be and that He has chosen me to be forever with Him. Though my light may dim, His becomes ever brighter. Though the path may seem hard, it will ease my heavy burden. One day I will leave this place, and He will welcome me into His eternal presence. I have the calling now, and I must not allow myself to doubt. I must welcome Him as much as He is willing to welcome me.

March 29

I spoke with my son regarding certain aspects of my employment. At work, they know that I have been having some memory issues. They don't yet know the extent of my concerns as I have not yet shared it with them. It's not as if I am hiding something, but at this time I do not know how things will develop. Having been a part-time faculty since 1985 and a full-time faculty since 1998, I don't remember any faculty member resigning because of this disease. I thought that I would not be contemplating retirement until my early 70's. That is not too unusual for an academic. Though the disease may be considered 'early onset,' I had not anticipated 'early retirement.' What a difference a diagnosis can make.

March 30

I won't have dreams. I won't have visions. I'll just be alive. I will be a life whose only purpose is to be alive. That is a very foreign idea to me. Having been a teacher of students spanning kindergarten through the doctoral level, I have always taught the need to have dreams and visions in one's life. To imagine a day where living is just being alive is unimaginable. The very essence of being human is to desire to grow and change.

From an early age, we teach our children to reach beyond themselves, to taste of their world and eventually to change it. It is one of the foundational beliefs of our humanity. We carry this belief into our adulthood and live it throughout our days. We don't abandon it because it is the very essence of being human.

We all believe that we have a purpose for living and it includes changing ourselves and others. Every hallmark of every life is the recognition of that change. Each child wants to find their own way. Each parent wants to help their child to be who they should be. Each teacher instructs to make a difference in the student. Each relationship is designed to make us grow. We learn in order to be aware and to succeed.

When these perspectives are interrupted, we lose a sense of our being. We just 'are' rather than 'are becoming.' The disease will move me to this point. My hope is that by that time I will have honored Him with all that He had given me to do.

March 31

I passed by a student on campus today who walked with a disfigured leg that caused him to swing it to the side a little. When I caught up with him, I said hi. He lifted his lowered head and smiled and said hi back. I then commented on the nice day, and he agreed.

How many times had he had this happen? How often did someone speak to him? Was he alone in his own infirmity and did not think that others wanted to join him?

I then thought of me and Alzheimer's. When will I be the one that others smile and say hi to? When will I be the one that they want to speak to? How often will I feel the need to just go back to my own world? Will they think of me like I thought of him, and will that be who I become?

I do not know the answers to these questions. But if you pass me along the way, be sure to say hi as I will need to raise my head and also have a great day. Even though you may leave me in my infirmity, know that you will have caused me to change a little bit that day.

April 7

Surprise! You don't have Alzheimer's! April fools!

If you had used me as the brunt of that April fools' joke, it would be seen as cruel. But if I say it about myself, it could be seen as a light-hearted way to deal with the situation. The reason for the latter is God. He has made us able to look at our own circumstances and find humor in them. Not that they aren't serious, but that we can see them as they truly are, only slight variations in the pathway to our eternity.

Humor is a gift that God has given to us to help us realize, in hard times, that His way is still easy and His burden is light. No other creature has this gift. They can act in funny ways, but they can't contemplate the humor in their difficulties. That is something that God has reserved for His image. We reflect His ways of looking at things and realize more clearly His will.

God gives to us many different ways to live through our situations. He comforts us, He is closer than a brother, He speaks to us, and He draws us near. I also believe that He has given to His image joy through humor. In so doing, we have the pleasure of honoring Him as we see that He is in complete control and that we can trust Him. If the trust that I have in Him in this situation can be seen through humor, then allow me to honor Him in it.

Today, I don't have Alzheimer's! April fools!

April 2

I went to fill up the coffee pot for tomorrow morning's coffee. I looked for the coffee measuring scoop and could not find it. I realized that it was not where it was supposed to be, but I had no idea where it could be. It wasn't as if I could not get my mind to remember, it was as if that individual fact never existed in my mind. I thought that I might have thrown it in the kitchen garbage, so I started to sift through the trash. To my surprise, while looking, I found a tablespoon from my everyday silverware set that I did not know I had thrown away, but no coffee scoop. I searched several of my kitchen drawers and found it in one where I would never have thought that I would have put it.

The amazing thing to me is that I am not talking about a lost memory when this happens, but I am looking to recall a real-life event that to me never actually happened. I didn't throw away the spoon, and I didn't misplace the coffee scoop. I know that I had to have done it because no one else is here. The interesting thing is that in all good conscience, that part of my memory could have testified in court that I had never done either thing. That is how completely the memory goes. I still have no memory of the loss, but I am glad that I will have fresh coffee in the morning.

April 4

Today I met with a publisher. I showed him examples of my work, and he offered me a book contract. He asked when I would be done, and I indicated in a couple of months or so. He liked that prospect, and we agreed to meet again then.

How amazing it is when God is in something. Last week I went online to just check on publishers. One of the names that popped up was this person. I sent an email, and the next day he responded. We set up a time, and now I am looking at the probability that you might be reading my writings because of that opportunity.

When things seem not to be going your way – after all, how else could you describe Alzheimer's? – God always shows through and the light at the end of the tunnel is a little brighter.

April 5

Cody, my dog, is getting older and has begun to have health issues. He once wanted to continually ride in the back of my Jeep and was always excited to jump in. These days, I have to grab his hind legs just after he leaps with the hope of getting him into the car. Sometimes our timing is off, and other times he doesn't jump high enough. That's when all 83 pounds of him ends up on the concrete floor of the garage and he is bewildered about what has just happened. This has begun to cause him to not always want to go for a ride, although he loves it.

It is hard to move beyond physical limitations. Just as with Cody, so many people have to live with this every day of their lives. They struggle to leap through the circumstances they encounter and sometimes end up in places they thought that they would never be. They know that God is there to lift them up, but sometimes it seems that He has just missed them. They are amazed at how many times they have not been able to overcome the situation. They, unlike Cody, know that it will most likely not change. Cody may try again, but they may never try again.

How does one face the realization that either now or one day in their life, they won't be able to 'work through it?' How can one live without ever doing or knowing again? How can a leap into thought end up in total darkness? That is a question to which I may never have an answer. I, like Cody, will look to those who love me for my reasons why and for my answers through the struggle.

April 7

I am watching them talk, I am listening to their conversation, but I don't remember the event they are talking about. I should know, but I am unable to focus my mind as the memory has gone. I do not remember and cannot make myself remember. I know the words they are saying and I understand that I should comprehend, but I am in a fog and their words do not aid me. I finally hear the words of their conversation that lead me to the place where I can begin to comprehend. They move closer to me in my mind, and I am able to grasp what I thought I did not know.

Slowly, the remembering has begun, and I find myself being surrounded by the memory and then suddenly in the memory. That is when I can see the thought because I now am part of the thought. It has found me, I have not found it. As if suddenly awakened and the mist has lifted, I am now in the glow of the thought and I know what I did not know and am able to see what I could not see.

April 8

I like the evening. Just me being me. I can relax, enjoy a movie, read a book, or watch a little TV. Being alone for me has never been thought of as being alone. I'm just doing things without someone else being around. But now, occasionally, I find that being alone is less comfortable. It's not as if I can't do the 'alone' things that I usually do, it's that I don't feel as comfortable being 'alone.'

I know that things are not really different, but my mind is still uneasy. The stillness becomes a little more uncomfortable and the silence a little more foreign. I am not afraid of someone or something else in the night, I am just a little afraid. I do not have the answer, but I feel as if I should. But how can you find an answer when the problem is not necessarily real but instead is in your mind?

That is a dilemma that I sometimes now face. That is a problem that I cannot yet solve. I must once again remember to trust Him, for He remains present when nothing else seems to be.

April 11

Today I left a phone message congratulating Katey, a friend's daughter, on her 45th birthday. I have known her since she was a little girl and have called her on her birthday for years. Her mother had already told her about the Alzheimer's. She talked with her mother indicating that she wanted to call me to thank me for my message but wondered what she should do. What if she had to leave a message for me and I could not remember that I had previously called her? Her mother told her to go ahead and contact me. After I heard her voice message on my phone, I let her mother know that her daughter had called. That is when the mother shared with me their conversation. I felt badly for Katey, as I could understand her concern and her desire not to put me in a position where I might not remember why she originally called.

This will continue to be an issue with others as I walk through my disease. The best way for them to help would be to treat me the way they would treat any other individual with a health problem. They need to realize that each day may be different and what was a case of memory loss yesterday may not be the case tomorrow. Just as if you were walking down the street with a handicapped person with braces on his legs. You would adjust your stride accordingly. Sometimes slower and other times faster. So it will be with me. Sometimes you might not have to trigger my memory, and at other times you may need to repeat the information as if I hadn't already known it.

This may not always be the case, and one day even I will wonder where my memory will be the next time I have to use it. But until then, we can walk and talk together, simply sharing our lives one with the other.

April 14

"I think, therefore I am." But what happens when I can no longer think? What happens when the disease robs me of my cognitive abilities? Do 'I' cease to exist?

When my mother lived with me, I learned about the differences in the stages of the disease. I watched her mind slowly forget little by little. Eventually, the general condition of her memory was limited to redeemable daily activities. She remembered some people, but not all. See could recognize some things from the past, but not all. She felt the continued joy of some situations, but not all. But when called upon to pray, she never showed the loss of a single understanding or occasion of the Lord's greatness and authority.

Her 'renewed mind,' given to her by God at her new birth, never faded. As she daily came closer to the time that she would be forever with Him, she never diminished in her mental capacity of knowing and loving Him. The old things of this world do pass away, but all things of the one to come live now and eternally in those called by His name. Though Momma and I forget, we will not be forgotten.

April 19

The graduate school had a modular course offered for students who are in the process of writing their dissertations. The graduate professors shared in scheduled sessions the different intentions for each chapter of the dissertation. My expertise is in formulating Chapter Two, the literature chapter. Although this was the first time since my diagnosis that I have taught this course, it seemed to me that no one felt as if I was not communicating to them what they needed to know. The session went fine, and the other professor who also taught in the session did not indicate any concern on his part.

I was glad that, when it was over, I could continue to feel confident in what I am supposed to do in my position. We have another full day tomorrow. I am hoping that, once again, all will go well. One day, I will have to let go of the place I have in the college, but I am glad that, at least to this point, I can continue on in the calling that the Lord has given to me.

April 25

I just returned from a four-day accreditation site visit. I, along with other faculty, evaluated the school to determine if it should continue in 'accredited' status. I was not sure that I wanted to go as I did not know what might happen relative to my memory. Would I not remember what I had just observed and therefore be unable to correctly discern the level of academic excellence of the school? I did not think that would be the case, but with a disease, one never knows for sure.

All things went well. They were reaccredited, and the team did a great job. I was glad that I had gone and that I was able to do what I needed to do. The day had not yet come where the disease would conquer my abilities in this arena. The Lord still has more for me to do. One day that may change, and I will need to recognize it. But today was not that day, and now is not that time.

April 30

Memory is an interesting thing. It is, it isn't, it stays, it fades, it lingers, it's lost, it was, it never has been. For me, memory has been all of these things. Alzheimer's has allowed me to experience memory through each of these facets. Of particular note is the last one: it never has been. This is the one most difficult to understand.

When I say that it never has been what I am saying is that the memory itself has completely disappeared. It's not that it has faded for a moment and that I can, through remembrance, bring it back again. Sometimes that does happen, but that is memory that was lost but has returned. It's also not memory that, if I look for it hard enough, will return. That is memory that faded but has come back. It's not memory that isn't and then is. That is memory that I can make myself recall. It is memory that I never had and I will never know again.

This is the memory that is hardest for people to understand. Surely, since they can remember, if I think about it hard enough, I should be able to remember. After all, I did it last time we thought about this memory. But this memory has now passed from my mind and no longer exists in my mind. I can't remember because it cannot be remembered. I have moved from having that memory to never having had that memory. It was at one time, but now, never has been.

May 4

I can remember that when I was a young child my family took a trip and ended up going to an amusement park and spending the day riding rides and playing at games. This particular park had a train where you could buy a ticket and then get onboard. The conductor would make his way through the different cars and collect the tickets and punch them and give them back. In that way, I felt that I belonged on the train and that he had confirmed the legitimacy of my presence. The ride continued and became one of the memorable moments of my youth.

Today, I am on a similar ride in life and await the conductor to come through and punch my ticket. It is not quite the same when you know that he has now entered your car. He smiles, walks past, and looks, and you smile back. He punches your ticket and indicates that you are off at the next stop. Not everyone's ticket gets punched, but you know that it is now your turn. Not everyone knows when their turn to depart will be, but you know that your time is soon. We all enjoy the ride, but for you, the ride has run its course.

The wait is not nearly as long as you thought it might be, and your Conductor will make sure that the departure is an easy one. He will be with you until you depart. He will show you which way to go next and to whom you are to show your punched ticket. The ride will have been an enjoyable one and the day in the park over. You will always remember the park, the ride, and the Conductor and find comfort in the fact that

He was always there and that He will always be there. And on that day, you will realize that the first ride with the Conductor will be over, but the next ride with Him will never end.

May 6

I cannot by faith say that I do not have Alzheimer's. I can by faith say that I can be healed of my Alzheimer's. These two phrases are sometimes confused with respect to believing what we think that God will do. God does heal. Some will say that God wants to heal us but that we, by our unbelief, don't allow Him to. I don't think that God is limited by anything, much less my unbelief. He may limit himself until I am willing to believe, but He is not limited to that either. He is sovereign, which means that He has absolute authority. His purposes cannot be altered by my unbelief. So, if I do believe, why am I not healed? That is simple. He is in charge of my life and works His will and purpose for me through my life.

The reasons for His purposes are many. For each of us they are different. We have no problem realizing that we all will not have the same job, calling, family, friends, etc. Each of these may be different, and how God orders our lives will bring about differences in every area, including in our healings. Some may never be healed, others may never be sick. Does one faith outshine the other? Some may do what we might call 'great things' for God, yet others just live for Him in each of the ordinary ways of life. Is the service of one greater than the service of the other? Is the first to believe greater than the last to believe? Is the one with the greater evidence of miracles more blessed than the one who sees God's blessings in the ordinary? We measure faith by the evidence of the movement of God. God measures faith as to how much we use our mustard seed.

Yes, God can heal. God does heal. We believe without a doubt that He will heal. But my confession is that I do have a disease and that God will do what He desires in my faith so that I can be, and yet may not be, healed. In this I have walked the walk of faith and have not doubted. I have merely put my faith in Him and not just in what He can do for me.

May 8

In my entrance hallway, there is a small table and an umbrella stand. When I go to vacuum, I put them both in the hallway closet and return them to their place after I have cleaned. Today, I returned the table but forgot to return the umbrella stand. When I looked at the finished hallway, I knew something was missing but could not remember what it might be. I stared at the table and tried to bring to my remembrance what I was trying to remember, but to no avail.

With Alzheimer's, I will sometimes know that something is not right but I may not have any idea of what that 'right' might be. Other times, such as this one, I will know that I 'should know' what it might be. I knew that something was missing and realized that I was conscious of that fact.

As I contemplated this, I then remembered that I had put something else in the closet. I opened the door and saw the umbrella stand. I immediately knew that this was the missing piece that would restore the previous familiar ambience to my hallway. I returned it, and everything was once again as before.

May 9

All along I have not been quite sure what I meant when I was talking about the 'fear.' I knew that it wasn't being afraid of something, but I wasn't clear as to what it meant. I think that I know now. It is the realization that I am not going to be able to live my life as I want, but rather it will be lived as the disease wants. The fear is not outside me but inside my mind as it realizes that it is beginning to know less and less of what it has known. I will be unaware of what I now know and will be less able to comprehend what I should know. My mind will fade as the disease increases. This is the picture of my fear. It is not the idea of being known; it is the idea of not knowing.

For to know is to be able to know that you are known. Though others may know you, if you cannot realize that, you remain unknown. This is the fear of being with others and yet being alone. This is the ultimate destination of Alzheimer's.

May 13

I received an invitation to a party the other day. I have been to the hosts' house a few times over the past couple of years. I know exactly where the house is located and exactly how to get there. But, as I looked at the text invitation, I could not remember how to get to their house. The invitation, being just a text, was not formal. It just listed the date and time, no location. Just 'their place.'

'Their place,' how casual and inviting, unless you're not sure where 'their place' is anymore. They don't yet know that I have Alzheimer's, so I can't easily indicate that I don't know how to get there. I could use my GPS and find the general location, but they didn't send directions in the text invitation. How do you find out where 'there' is if you don't want anyone to know that you don't know where 'there' is? Having Alzheimer's and not letting it show becomes more and more difficult each day.

I texted back and said 'no' to the invitation. Didn't offer a real reason for not coming, just said 'no.' It became one more party that I was unable to attend.

May 14

Today is Mother's Day. I remember my mom and her time with Alzheimer's. She faced it with such grace and peace. She never became bitter or even lost her sense of humor. She, like me, knew she had the disease but did not let the disease prevent her from being herself, as long as she could. She laughed and enjoyed life through every day that God gave her. She knew her condition until the last but did not let it affect her disposition. She thanked God for each day and her time in it. I watched with amazement her resting in the Lord despite the circumstances.

She never had a bad day, just days that she lived as if they had meaning beyond the circumstances in which she found herself. Her example guides me and helps me to see the truth in my circumstances. Life is to be lived to the fullest. Each day has its moments of excellence where we can touch other lives and help them to see more clearly. As each day gives clearer meaning to the significance of life, the opportunity to demonstrate that significance in small ways presents itself. In this manner, we not only continue to live, we teach others how to continue to live. Each example of courage becomes an example of strength for others to follow. In this way, a diminishing life can actually impact the future of someone else's life. My mother did this for me. I can only hope that I can do the same for others.

May 17

I am beginning to relate to II Timothy 1:7, where the Word proclaims that, "God hath not given us a spirit of fear, but of power, and of love, and of a sound mind." Though I knew the verse by heart, it had never occurred to me that the words power, love, and sound mind would be used together in such a way. Most people, including me, don't think of them as connecting. Power and love are not generally connected with a sound mind. Fear is many times seen as lack of faith, not lack of power, love, and a sound mind. If it had said 'imagined fear,' that would have made more sense, because in our minds we many times imagine all kinds of things that are not true. It says a spirit of fear. An actual thing that creates fear. That makes it not only wrestling for one's mind, it makes it wrestling for one's mind in the spirit realm.

When one moves into the spiritual realm, many kinds of combinations can exist. That is because we each have different areas in which we are stronger and weaker than others. We deal with those areas that we are weak in so that He can be made strong. In this way, God makes us strong as He has given to us a spirit that can deal with these forces in our spiritual nature. It is not just to have power or to have love or to have a sound mind, it is to be able to then overcome the spirit of fear that would try to weaken us in these resolves.

Though we may be weak in any of these three areas, we can believe and rely upon God's Word to strengthen us in our resolve to live in the Spirit and to proclaim by faith these principals. Not blindly, but knowing through His Word that He has spoken it and that He will be with us as we endeavor to live it. Even when I will not be unable to realize it, it will be the Holy Spirit, and not a spirit of fear, that will show though me the simplicity of His Truth.

May 19

I have to think about what I will say after I have thought about what I did say. What an unusual phrase to use when thinking about general conversation. The mind thinks so many times just as part of the interactions we have with each other. We do not have to coax it or cause it to think. It just does. But when you are thinking, the mind relies on stored memories and situations to draw from in order to become a part of the conversation. But what if you do not completely control the thinking? What if the mind does not put all the pieces together correctly? You are thinking and then interacting and then wondering why you said what you just said. Was it right or not, did it fit into the conversation, did you make sense? How do you continue in the conversation after you may have completely missed it without knowing that you have? This is a conundrum I am beginning to face.

I speak because my mind tells me I know, but then I realize that I do not. The people I am speaking with may not always see this, as I, like most of us do when we have missed the point, correct myself. The difference is that the correction is sometimes also a gamble. If presented well, it is just seen as normal corrective conversation. But if not corrected soon enough, the others in the conversation must correct me. At this point, that correction seems normal to them, but I wonder when it will no longer seem that way. When will my thoughts of error and of inappropriate connections become too obvious to others? That day will come, as so many others will. But I hope that I will be the first to see it.

Final

Today, you have read my mind. Tomorrow, it may not be there. All that I have said has value only if it echoes the words of my Lord. If not, my truths presented are as sounding brass and tinkling symbols.

My life is not the value, His life in me is what gives it value. My death is not the payment, His death is the everlasting sacrifice. I will live not because I am, I will live because He is the I am. He is the Alpha and Omega, the beginning and the end. I only came to be because He first knew me. He will live forever. I will live in Him forever. My time is not measured by my greatness. My time will be measured in how greatly I have followed Him.

What is 'this' man that thou art mindful of Him? How great are your mercies to those whom you love! Your love is from everlasting to everlasting toward those who fear You, and Your righteousness is with their children's children. How wonderful are Your works! The Lord Himself has authored my life, and that is marvelous in my eyes.

About the Author

Timothy D. Norton lived in Virginia Beach, Virginia, before coming to ORU as an undergraduate vocal performance major. After graduation, he taught music at Rock Church Academy in Virginia Beach and later served as its Principal. During this time, he also taught humanities in ORU's online evening extension program.

When ORU's Graduate School of Education started its Summer Institute, Tim regularly came back to Tulsa to teach as a part of the program. In 1998, ORU invited Dr. Norton to teach full-time in the School of Education's graduate program, a position he still holds today.

Dr. Norton has a Bachelor of Arts in Music from Oral Roberts University, a Master of Arts in Education from Regent University, an Educational Specialist degree from The College of William and Mary in Virginia and a Doctorate of Education from the College of William and Mary in Virginia.

He currently resides in Tulsa, Oklahoma.

www.ingramcontent.com/pod-product-compliance
Lightning Source LLC
Chambersburg PA
CBHW031416250726
48656CB00002B/706